Kids

Asthma

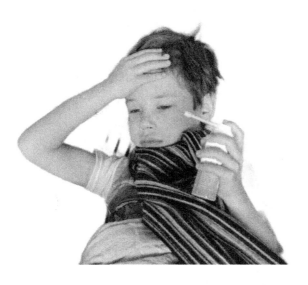

A Complete Guide to Healing Asthma in Children - Symptoms Diagnosis, Triggers and Allergy Management, Treatment Options, and Lifestyle Adjustment for Effective Control, Relief, Cure.

Dr. George K. Shelley

CONCLUSION

BOOKS BY THE AUTHOR

INTRODUCTION

An Inhalation of Life

Every life is a different story, a collection of experiences that mold who we are. These experiences might be commonplace or remarkable, happy or difficult, but they are always incredibly human. In these pages, I welcome you inside the most intimate and transforming chapter of my life, a narrative that centers around a simple, yet significant act: breathing.

I have committed my life as Dr. George K. Shelley to the practice of medicine and the advancement of knowledge. My professional life has been an examination of the intricate workings of the human body, a never-ending quest to understand how we function, why we suffer, and how we recover. Despite the fact that my professional life has been defined by my clinical training and scientific knowledge, it was a personal journey that would open my eyes to the genuine depth and wonder of the human experience.

It started in the dead of winter, in the heart of our family. Daniel, my son, was only four years old when he was diagnosed with asthma. A cool afternoon had given way to a nice evening spent in front of the fireplace, which provided a soft heat for the entire house. Daniel's jovial laughter echoed the purity and energy of boyhood as the evening progressed. I was unaware at the time that this special occasion would usher in a significant turning point in our lives.

The laughter that had previously permeated our house abruptly gave place to a far more unsettling cough and strained breathing. As I hugged my kid close, I felt a wave of panic go over me, and I knew something terrible had happened. In that instant, I first realized the humbling force of vulnerability and the sorrow a parent feels as they watch their kid suffer. Daniel, my beloved son, was having trouble breathing.

The entire night was clouded by anxiety and constant watchfulness. Daniel was immediately diagnosed with asthma in the hospital, which would later become a constant companion in our lives. I will never forget seeing his little, frail body attached to nebulizers and inhalers, the ritualistic intake of corticosteroids and albuterol becoming what would make us who we were.

I would later discover that asthma is a disorder that affects everyone equally. It is a disorder that has no regard for an individual's age, gender, or socioeconomic standing. It may hit with the finesse of wind or the ferocity of a storm, upsetting lives and changing the narratives of people who experience it. I had studied asthma in the abstract as a doctor, but as a father, I would get to know it deeply and viscerally.

The odyssey that took place following Daniel's diagnosis was evidence of both the never-ending depths of human resiliency and the ceaseless search for knowledge. It was a journey characterized by a parent's steadfast love, a family's cooperation, and the direction of committed medical experts.

We started along the road of comprehending, coping with, and ultimately flourishing with asthma together.

Over the years, we overcame difficulties ranging from restless nights and absences from school to unpleasant difficulties with medication administration and the constant worry about asthma attacks. But for every difficulty we overcame, there was a triumphant moment, a chance for development, and a realization of the incredible power of the human spirit.

The outcome of our journey, one that is shared by countless parents and caregivers who walk in the shoes of children with asthma, is this book. It is a voyage of knowledge, empowerment, and optimism. It is evidence of children's resiliency and the enduring commitment of their parents and caregivers.

We shall dig into the details of pediatric asthma in the chapters that follow, from comprehending the condition's basics to identifying its symptoms and causes. We'll talk about the confusing world of drugs, the necessity of building asthma-friendly surroundings, and the vital support system that we, as caregivers, must establish.

Although my own experience is interwoven across these pages, it is not the only story. Instead, it serves as a common thread in each of our individual stories—those of parents and other caregivers who overcame the difficulties brought on by pediatric asthma every day with courage, tenacity, and optimism. It is a theme that emphasizes the fortitude of kids who not only successfully control their asthma but also thrive in the face of its difficulties.

But this book is for everyone who wants knowledge, insight and hope, not only those who have traveled this route. It is for the medical professionals who devote their entire careers to treating children with asthma as well as the dedicated researchers who are delving into the complexities of this illness. It is for the teachers, friends, and extended family who offer asthmatic children essential assistance.

The path of pediatric asthma is a shared one, replete with the inspiration that results from resiliency, the hope that results from knowledge, and the strength that results from understanding. It is my goal that you will find the inspiration and direction you need in these pages to turn the difficulties associated with asthma into opportunities and to realize the limitless potential that each kid, parent, and caregiver possesses.

I urge you to go on a trip that is both personal and universal as you read this book. This journey will highlight the remarkable power of the human spirit. The voyage embraces the heart and spirit of the human experience, transcending clinical knowledge and medical textbooks.

In the end, it's not simply a book about childhood asthma; it's a book about the astonishing power of the human spirit to breathe comfortably and embrace life's limitless possibilities.

With warm regards,

Dr. George K. Shelley

Chapter 1

Understanding Kids' Asthma

Asthma is a complicated and sometimes challenging health condition, especially in children. Let's explore the world of childhood asthma by learning about what it is, how prevalent it is, the serious effects it may have on kids' health, and the common symptoms and triggers that parents and other caregivers should be aware of.

What is Asthma?

Asthma is a chronic respiratory condition that damages the lungs' airways. These bronchial tubes, which are also known as airways, are in charge of transferring air into and out of the lungs. These airways become inflamed, swollen, and sensitive in an asthmatic individual. The airways become more constricted as a result of the inflammation, making it harder for air to enter and exit easily.

Asthma has a propensity to flare up and produce abrupt symptoms, which are sometimes referred to as asthma attacks or episodes. The muscles around the airways tighten, the lining of the airways swells even more, and excessive mucus is generated during an asthma attack. These modifications cause a restricted and narrowed airway, which makes it challenging for the affected person to breathe.

Asthma is a chronic illness, so it never completely goes away, but with the appropriate approach to therapy and lifestyle changes, its symptoms may be managed and controlled. It's critical to realize that asthma can be controlled and that those who have it—including kids— may have full and active lives with the right treatment.

The Airway's Role in Breathing

Let's look more closely at the role of the airways in breathing to better comprehend asthma. Air enters the trachea (windpipe) and bronchial tubes through the nose as we breathe in. Like the limbs of a tree, these tubes, or airways, spread out into the lungs and become progressively narrower. These airways in a healthy person let air enter and exit easily, allowing optimal oxygen exchange.

Inflammation and Narrowing

In asthma, the airways become inflamed, which causes swelling and more mucus to produce. The airways become more constricted and more sensitive as a result of the inflammation. These triggers can cause the muscles that surround the airways to contract, further constricting the airway. The hallmark symptoms of asthma, including wheezing, coughing, shortness of breath, and tightness in the chest, are brought on by the simultaneous effects of inflammation and muscle constriction.

Prevalence and Impact on Children's Health

The frequency of asthma has been progressively increasing over the past few decades, especially among children. Asthma is a global health concern. The Centers for Disease Control and Prevention (CDC) estimate that 1 in 13 Americans in the country have asthma and that this number rises to 1 in 12 for children.

The effects of asthma on kids' health are extensive and varied:

Missed School Days

Children with asthma frequently have symptoms that might make it difficult for them to go about their everyday lives, including going to school. Missed school days due to frequent asthma attacks and hospitalizations may have an impact on a child's academic performance and social development.

Reduced Physical Activity

Physical activity is essential for the growth and development of a child. Asthma, however, can restrict a child's capacity to engage in physical activity, which can result in a decline in fitness and general health.

Sleep Disruption

The symptoms of asthma, such as coughing and breathing problems, tend to get worse at night. Both the kids and the parents' sleep patterns may be affected, which will lower their general well-being and quality of life.

Emotional Impact

Children who have a chronic illness like asthma may experience emotional stress. Regarding their symptoms or the requirement for medicine and medical procedures, they could feel worry, frustration, or anxiety.

Medical Bills

Families affected by asthma may also have financial difficulties. Parents and other caregivers may be financially burdened by the price of prescriptions, medical appointments, and ER trips.

Individual Variability

It's critical to understand that every child has a unique set of asthma triggers. One child may not be affected by what causes symptoms in another. The key to managing a child's asthma is to identify their unique triggers and take preventative or control measures.

Factors Influencing Prevalence

The prevalence of asthma in children is influenced by a number of variables. Children who have a family history of asthma or allergies are more likely to acquire the ailment, so genetics does play a part. Children's chances of developing asthma can also be increased by environmental factors such as exposure to cigarette smoke, air pollution, and allergens.

Causes and Risk Factors

In order to effectively treat this complicated respiratory disorder, it is essential to understand the causes and risk factors of pediatric asthma. Let's examine the many facets of childhood asthma, including its hereditary and familial components, environmental impacts, the function of allergens, the hygiene theory, and the substantial negative effects of air pollution on asthmatic children.

Genetic Factors and Family History

Genetic Predisposition

A kid is more likely to acquire asthma if there is a family history of the ailment since asthma frequently includes a hereditary component. Several significant genetic variables contribute to the development of asthma, despite the fact that it is a complicated illness impacted by several genes.

Family History of Asthma

A child is more likely to acquire asthma if one or both of its parents do. In fact, compared to children without asthmatic parents, children with one asthmatic parent had a 25% higher chance of having asthma. The risk is significantly higher if both parents suffer from asthma.

Specific Genetic Markers

A number of unique genetic markers linked to asthma risk have been found by researchers. These biomarkers are linked to immune system activity, airway inflammation, and airway responsiveness. Studies on the genetics of asthma have shed light on its basic causes and suggested new therapy options.

Gene-Environment Interactions

It's crucial to understand that genetics do not account for all cases of asthma. Gene-environment interactions are very important. In those who are genetically susceptible to asthma, environmental factors such as exposure to allergens and pollution can influence the development and progression of asthma.

The Environmental Connection

Environmental factors have an equivalent impact on asthma susceptibility as hereditary ones do. These elements can cause asthma symptoms, exacerbate the illness, or even hasten the onset of the condition in people with genetic predispositions.

Common Environmental Factors

1. **Allergens:** Children who are sensitive to certain allergens, such as pollen, dust mites, pet dander, and mold, may experience asthmatic symptoms.

2. **Respiratory Infections:** Viral respiratory infections, particularly in infancy, might raise the chance of developing asthma or exacerbate pre-existing asthma.

3. **Tobacco Smoke:** Exposure to secondhand smoke is a substantial risk factor for

pediatric asthma, both during pregnancy and after birth.

4. **Air Pollution:** Pollutants including particulate matter and ozone, which define poor air quality, can irritate the airways and aggravate asthma symptoms.

5. **Occupational Exposures:** Children are more at risk if their parents or other caregivers bring allergens home accidentally from work where they are exposed to compounds that cause asthma.

6. **Early Antibiotic Use:** According to some studies, using antibiotics often and early in a child's life may raise their chance of developing asthma.

7. **Dietary Factors:** Pregnancy and early childhood diet may affect the chance of developing asthma. For instance, eating a

lot of fruits and vegetables may be beneficial.

The Complex Interaction

It is complicated how genetics and environmental factors interact to cause asthma. Environmental exposures can either cause asthma attacks or act as a preventative measure, but genetics lays the setting for vulnerability. For management and prevention, it is essential to comprehend these relationships.

Allergies and Their Role in Childhood Asthma

Asthma and allergies commonly coexist. Asthma symptoms can be triggered or made worse by allergic responses, which are common in children with asthma. The allergy-asthma connection refers to this strong association between allergies and asthma.

Common Allergens in Childhood Asthma

1. **Pollen:** Hay fever or allergic rhinitis, seasonal pollen allergies, can make children's asthma symptoms worse.

2. **Dust Mites:** Allergens from dust mites are frequently used as asthma and allergy triggers. Bedding, upholstered furniture, and carpets are ideal habitats for dust mites.

3. **Pet Allergens:** For those who are allergic or asthmatic, proteins in pet dander, saliva, and urine can act as allergens.

4. **Mold:** Mold spores, which are frequently present in moist conditions, can cause allergic responses as well as asthmatic symptoms.

5. **Cockroach Allergens:** Exposure to cockroach allergens, which are frequently present in urban settings, can lead to the onset and worsening of asthma.

6. **Food Allergies:** Although gastrointestinal problems are the main symptom of food allergies, some kids may also develop asthma as a side effect of an allergic response.

The Atopic March

The term "atopic march," which reflects the usual pattern of allergic disease development, commonly beginning with eczema in infancy, followed by allergic rhinitis (hay fever), and finally asthma, is sometimes used to describe the passage from allergies to asthma. Although not all people with allergies will acquire asthma, those who have a family history of the disease are more likely to do so.

Immunoglobulin E (IgE) Antibodies

Immunoglobulin E (IgE) antibodies are important in the relationship between allergies and asthma. A person's immune system produces IgE antibodies in response to exposure to an allergen to which they are sensitized, causing allergic responses and asthma symptoms. Anti-IgE antibody medications help control severe allergic asthma by lowering IgE levels.

The Hygiene Hypothesis

The Paradox of Cleanliness

The hygiene theory investigates the discrepancy between improved cleanliness and the growing incidence of autoimmune and allergic disorders, particularly asthma.

It implies that decreased exposure to certain bacteria throughout childhood brought on by better hygienic practices may raise the likelihood of allergies and asthma.

The Role of Early Microbial Exposure

According to the hygiene hypothesis, a child's immune system develops significantly as a result of early microbial encounters. The immune system learns to discriminate between dangerous infections and innocuous things, such as pollen or pet dander, by exposure to a variety of bacteria in the environment. Absent such exposure, an excessively sensitive immune system may result in allergies and asthma.

Supporting Evidence

The discovery that children who grow up in more rural or farm surroundings, where they are exposed to a greater diversity of microorganisms, have lower incidences of asthma and allergies, lends support to the hygiene theory. On the other hand, children who grow up in metropolitan and highly sterilized settings may be more susceptible to allergies and asthma.

Balancing Cleanliness and Microbial Exposure

The hygiene hypothesis does not support unsanitary settings, despite emphasizing the significance of microbial exposure. Sanitation and good hygiene habits, such as hand washing, are still crucial for avoiding infectious infections. Finding a balance between maintaining cleanliness and giving kids some exposure to various bacteria, however, can be advantageous for the growth of their immune systems.

The Impact of Air Pollution on Children with Asthma

A Looming Threat

Children who already have asthma are in serious danger from air pollution, which worsens their symptoms and raises the possibility that they may develop asthma. It is becoming more urgent to address the effects of air pollution on respiratory health as urbanization and industry progress.

Common Air Pollutants

Children who have asthma are known to be impacted by a number of common air pollutants:

1. **Particulate Matter (PM):** PM is made up of minute airborne particles including dust, soot, and allergies. PM can enter the lungs deeply and aggravate asthma symptoms.

2. **Ground-Level Ozone:** A component of smog, ground-level ozone can irritate the airways and exacerbate asthma symptoms. It can cause serious respiratory irritation.

3. **Nitrogen Dioxide (NO2):** Nitrogen Dioxide (NO2) is a pollutant that is created through combustion processes, such as those seen in industrial settings and motor vehicles. It can impair lung function and exacerbate asthma symptoms.

4. **Sulfur Dioxide (SO2):** When sulfur-containing fossil fuels are burned, SO2 is released into the atmosphere. It may aggravate asthma by irritating the airways.

5. **Volatile Organic Compounds (VOCs):** VOCs are emitted from a variety of sources, such as building supplies and home goods.

They may exacerbate asthma symptoms and add to indoor air pollution.

The Vulnerability of Children

Children who have asthma are more susceptible to the negative effects of air pollution. They frequently breathe more quickly than adults do, increasing their exposure to toxins, and their growing lungs are more prone to injury. Long-term exposure to air pollution may deteriorate asthma management, increase the frequency of asthma attacks, and eventually impair lung function.

The Role of Location

Depending on the region, air pollution may have different effects on children's asthma. Children who reside in high air pollution places, such as urban cores, industrial zones, or close to major highways, may experience more difficulties with asthma.

Protecting Children from Air Pollution

Improving air quality regulations, lowering emissions from cars and other industrial sources, and promoting sustainable energy alternatives are all actions taken to safeguard children from the damaging impacts of air pollution. Parents and other caregivers who care for children should also take measures to reduce their exposure to indoor pollutants and keep an eye on the air quality in their surroundings.

We have looked at the several root causes and danger signs of pediatric asthma. A child's predisposition to developing asthma is influenced by genetics and family history, and it may also be triggered or made worse by environmental factors such as exposure to allergens, respiratory infections, cigarette smoke, and air pollution. The allergy-asthma connection emphasizes the part allergens play in the emergence of asthma, while the hygiene theory emphasizes the significance of early microbial exposure in immune system formation. Finally, the severe negative effects of air pollution on asthmatic children highlight the necessity of taking environmental protection measures to safeguard respiratory health.

Healthcare professionals, parents, caregivers, and educators must comprehend these causes and risk factors. It enables well-informed choices, preventative measures, and efficient management techniques to provide asthmatic kids the assistance they need to live healthy lives.

Our goal as we move through this thorough manual is to arm you with the information and resources required to deal with the difficulties presented by childhood asthma, enabling you to give every child the support and care they need to breathe easily and look forward to a future full of limitless opportunities.

Chapter 2

Diagnosis and Early Intervention

articularly in children, asthma is a disorder that needs prompt diagnosis and intervention. A child's chances of managing symptoms, avoiding complications, and ensuring that they live a long and meaningful life are all improved the sooner asthma is detected and managed. Here, we'll talk about how important it is to spot asthma symptoms in kids, comprehend the value of early detection, and form a working relationship with medical staff.

Recognizing the Signs of Asthma in Children

Because asthma symptoms might be mistaken for those of other respiratory disorders, especially in young children who might not be able to express their discomfort properly, it can be difficult to spot the symptoms of asthma in children. As a result, it's crucial for parents and other caregivers to keep an eye out for any changes in their child's health. The following are some typical symptoms of asthma in kids:

1. **Frequent Coughing:** Asthma symptoms might include persistent coughing, especially at night or in the morning. This cough might be dry or mucus-producing.

2. **Wheezing:** When your child breaths, especially during exhale, a high-pitched whistling sound is made. It frequently serves as a glaring sign of constricted airways.

3. **Shortness of Breath:** If your kid frequently has shortness of breath, particularly during play or physical exercise, it may be an asthmatic symptom. They could seem to be having trouble breathing.

4. **Chest Tightness:** Some asthmatic kids report feeling tight or uncomfortable in their chests. They could find this experience upsetting.

5. **Nighttime Symptoms:** Asthma symptoms frequently get worse at night. Asthma may be a factor if your kid complains of

coughing, wheezing, or having trouble breathing when they first wake up.

6. **Frequent Respiratory Infections:** Children with asthma may appear to get colds or respiratory infections more frequently than their peers. This is a result of their more sensitive and prone to inflammatory airways.

7. **Increased Mucus Production:** Asthma can cause the airways to produce more mucus, which can make it harder to breathe and cause coughing.

8. **Reduced Physical Activity:** Some asthmatic kids may avoid sports and exercise because of their symptoms, which can have a negative impact on their fitness and ability to participate in activities they like.

It's crucial to remember that not all children with asthma may have all of these symptoms, and that symptom intensity might change. While some kids may only occasionally exhibit symptoms, others could do so more regularly.

The Importance of Early Diagnosis

Effective asthma care, especially in children, starts with early diagnosis. What's the significance of early diagnosis?

1. **Better Symptom Control:** By treating your child's asthma symptoms efficiently as soon as they are identified, you can lessen the frequency and intensity of asthma attacks.

2. **Prevention of Complications:** problems that can be avoided include lung damage and long-term problems from uncontrolled

asthma. Early intervention can help prevent these kinds of issues.

3. **Improved Quality of Life:** Children with asthma who are properly controlled can enjoy active, happy lives. A key component of doing this is early diagnosis.

4. **Reduced Emergency Room Visits:** The frequency of visits to the emergency room caused by severe asthma attacks can be decreased by prompt diagnosis and treatment.

5. **Less Missed School and Activities:** If your child's asthma is properly managed, they can participate in sports, school, and other activities without being frequently interrupted.

6. **Peace of Mind:** An early diagnosis enables parents and other caregivers to

take proactive measures to ensure their child's well-being by giving them a clear understanding of their condition.

Working with Healthcare Professionals

It's crucial to get a professional medical evaluation and advice if you think your child might have asthma based on the symptoms you've noticed. Here are some tips on how to collaborate with medical experts to diagnose and treat your child's asthma:

1. **Consult Your Pediatrician:** The first place to go for an asthma evaluation is typically your child's primary care physician, who is often a pediatrician. Discuss your worries and observations with the pediatrician, who will perform a complete evaluation.

2. **Medical History:** Your child's doctor will ask about his or her medical background, including any allergies or asthma in the family. Be ready to offer this data when asked.

3. **Physical Examination:** A physical examination will be done by the healthcare provider, who may also listen for wheezing or other unusual lung sounds.

4. **Lung Function Tests:** Spirometry or other lung function tests may be carried out if asthma is suspected. These examinations gauge how well your child can breathe in and out.

5. **Allergy Testing:** In order to determine potential allergens that might be causing your child's asthma symptoms, allergy testing may be advised.

6. **Peak Flow Monitoring:** Peak flow monitoring can be used to assess how well the lungs of older kids are working. For monitoring the control of asthma, this can be a helpful tool.

7. **Establish an Asthma Action Plan:** Create an asthma action plan in collaboration with the healthcare practitioner for your kid. This strategy covers what to do in a variety of circumstances, such as asthma attacks.

8. **Medication Management:** If asthma is identified in your kid, the doctor will talk to you about your choices for treating it, which may include using nebulizers or inhalers to provide medication. Make sure you are aware of the proper usage of these devices.

9. **Regular Follow-Ups:** Managing asthma is a continuous procedure. Make routine

follow-up meetings with your child's doctor to check on their development and modify the treatment plan as necessary.

10. **Open Communication:** Retain an honest and open line of contact with your child's doctor. Share any symptoms or concerns right away.

Navigating Diagnostic Challenges

Diagnosing childhood asthma can be problematic owing to the overlap of symptoms with other respiratory illnesses and the variety of asthma presentations. Differential diagnosis is the practice of separating asthma from other medical illnesses that have similar symptoms.

Conditions That May Mimic Asthma

1. **Respiratory Infections:** Respiratory infections, such as viral bronchitis or pneumonia, can cause symptoms similar to asthma, including coughing and wheezing.

2. **Gastroesophageal Reflux Disease (GERD):** GERD can lead to acid reflux into the airways, generating cough and asthma-like symptoms.

3. **Vocal Cord Dysfunction (VCD):** VCD is a disorder where the vocal cords constrict during inhalation, leading to wheezing and shortness of breath that can mimic asthma.

4. **Congenital Heart Defects:** Some congenital heart defects can present with symptoms resembling asthma, such as shortness of breath and chest tightness.

5. **Cystic Fibrosis:** Cystic fibrosis may induce respiratory symptoms comparable to asthma, including coughing and wheezing.

The Role of Clinical Evaluation

A complete clinical evaluation, including medical history, physical examination, lung function tests, and, where appropriate, specialist testing, is critical in separating asthma from other illnesses. Collaboration among pediatricians, pulmonologists, allergists, and other healthcare specialists may be essential to establish an appropriate diagnosis.

It's vital to remember that every child is unique, and asthma can appear differently in each individual. Therefore, an individualized approach to diagnosis and treatment is crucial to provide the greatest outcomes for your kid.

Diagnosing children's asthma needs a joint effort between doctors, healthcare professionals, parents, and caregivers. Pediatricians play a vital role in the initial examination, whereas lung function tests give objective data on lung function. Allergy testing helps identify possible triggers, and maintaining an asthma diary benefits in tracking symptoms and therapy. Differential diagnosis is required to rule out other illnesses with similar symptoms. With a comprehensive and evidence-based diagnostic approach, children with asthma can receive the treatment and support they need to manage their illness effectively and enjoy healthy lives.

Chapter 3

Asthma Triggers and Allergens: Preventing Asthma Attacks

Asthma symptoms in children can be induced or aggravated by different variables in their surroundings. For successful management of these asthma triggers, understanding and identification are essential. Here, we'll look at how to manage allergens to lessen asthma symptoms, examine common asthma triggers in homes and settings, and offer advice on how to make your home more asthma-friendly.

Identifying Common Triggers in the Home and Environment

The term "asthma trigger" refers to things or situations that might irritate the airways and cause or exacerbate asthma symptoms. Although triggers might differ from child to child, some are more frequently seen in indoor and outdoor settings. You should be aware of the following common asthma triggers:

1. **Allergens:** Allergens are chemicals that can make people with asthma experience allergic responses. Pollen, dust mites, pet hair, mold spores, and cockroach droppings are examples of common allergies. Inflammation of the airways brought on by allergic responses can exacerbate asthma symptoms.

2. **Tobacco Smoke:** Smoke from tobacco products, whether inhaled actively or passively (secondhand smoke), is a significant asthma trigger. Smoke irritates the airways, which causes more inflammation and symptoms of asthma.

3. **Air Pollution:** The symptoms of asthma can be made worse by outdoor air pollution, which includes pollutants including fine particulate matter (PM2.5), ozone, and nitrogen dioxide. Gas stoves and fireplaces are two common sources of indoor air pollution that can be troublesome.

4. **Respiratory Infections:** Viral respiratory illnesses like the flu or the common cold can cause asthma attacks. Children with asthma must be protected against and treated for respiratory infections.

5. **Exercise:** While being physically active is good for general health, some kids with asthma may have a condition called exercise-induced bronchoconstriction (EIB), in which doing so brings on asthma symptoms. However, the majority of kids with asthma can engage in physical activities safely with the right care.

6. **Stress and Emotional Factors:** Anxiety and emotional stress can occasionally cause or exacerbate asthma symptoms. Managing stress and offering children emotional support are essential components of managing asthma.

7. **Weather Changes:** For some children with asthma, cold, dry air as well as abrupt weather changes might be triggers. Making sure your child is dressed correctly for the climate will help reduce these triggers.

8. **Strong Odors and Irritants:** The airways can get irritated by strong aromas from perfumes, cleaning supplies, and other chemicals. When feasible, try to use fragrance-free or low-odor products.

9. **Pests and Pest Allergens:** Rodents and their allergens, such as cockroach droppings, can be serious asthma triggers. In order to eliminate these allergies in the house, effective pest control techniques are required.

Managing Allergens to Reduce Asthma Symptoms

One of the most important aspects of managing asthma is minimizing exposure to asthma triggers. To aid children with asthma symptoms, the following management techniques for common allergens and triggers are provided:

1. **Allergen-Proof Bedding:** To stop dust mites and other allergens from gathering in bedding, cover mattresses, pillows, and box springs with allergen-proof coverings.

2. **Regular Cleaning:** Regular cleaning can help lower allergy levels in the house. Use a vacuum cleaner with a HEPA filter to frequently vacuum upholstered furniture, carpets, and rugs.

3. **Reduce Humidity:** Humid conditions are ideal for mold and dust mites. To keep interior humidity levels between 30 and 50%, use a dehumidifier.

4. **Wash Bedding:** To eliminate dust mites, wash bedding, including sheets and pillows, once a week in hot water (130°F or higher).

5. **Minimize Pet Allergens:** If your child is allergic to pets and you have them, you might want to take precautions like keeping them out of bedrooms and utilizing high-efficiency air purifiers.

6. **Quitting Smoking:** In order to safeguard your child with asthma, it's crucial that all smokers in the home give up their cigarettes or make their home smoke-free.

7. **Proper Ventilation:** To lessen indoor air pollution, make sure your house has enough ventilation by utilizing exhaust fans in the kitchen and bathroom and opening windows when you can.

8. **Regular Pest Control:** Reduce cockroach and rodent allergies by quickly addressing pest problems with expert pest control services.

9. **Avoidance of Strong Odors:** Use cleaning products without strong odors or those with a milder aroma.

Creating an Asthma-Friendly Home

Making your house an asthma-friendly space is a proactive move toward successfully controlling your child's asthma. Here are some more ideas to make your house asthma-friendly:

1. **Asthma Action Plan Display:** Display the child's asthma action plan in a prominent spot that is simple to get to inside the home. This serves to remind family members and caregivers what to do in the event of an asthma emergency.

2. **Medication Management/Accessibility:** Make sure you and your kid understand how to use inhalers or nebulizers

properly and keep asthma medications easily available. Everyone in the home should be able to locate it.

3. **Smoke-Free Environment:** Strictly enforce the no-smoking rule within the home. Make sure that nobody smokes indoors or near places where kids congregate.

4. **Allergen Control:** As previously noted, take measures to lessen allergens such as dust mites, pollen, and pet dander. Regular cleaning, appropriate ventilation, and the use of air purifiers are all part of this.

5. **Healthy Lifestyle:** Encourage your family to lead a healthy lifestyle that includes a balanced diet, frequent exercise, and stress management methods.

6. **Regular Check-Ups:** Set up routine follow-up meetings with your child's doctor to check their asthma and modify their treatment plan as necessary.

7. **Asthma Education:** As your child gets older, include them in controlling their illness by teaching them about asthma.

You may dramatically lessen the negative effects of asthma triggers on your child's health and help them live a more comfortable and symptom-free life by implementing these methods and making your house an asthma-friendly environment.

Vaccinations and Asthma Prevention

The Role of Vaccinations in Asthma Prevention

Asthma exacerbations in children can be brought on by respiratory infections, which are significantly decreased by vaccinations.

Key Vaccinations for Asthma Prevention:

1. **Influenza (Flu) Vaccine:** All kids, especially those with asthma, should get the yearly flu shot. Children with asthma who contract influenza infections may experience severe respiratory symptoms.

2. **Pneumococcal Vaccine:** The pneumococcal vaccination aids in preventing infections brought on by the bacteria Streptococcus pneumoniae, which can aggravate asthma.

3. **Tdap Vaccine:** The Tdap vaccine guards against whooping cough, tetanus, and diphtheria. Long-lasting coughing fits

brought on by pertussis might resemble asthma symptoms.

Importance of Vaccination:

In addition to lowering the risk of respiratory infections, vaccination also lessens the possibility that these illnesses would result in asthma attacks. An essential preventative approach in the management of asthma in children is to make sure they get all of their vaccines.

The Importance of Regular Check-Ups

Monitoring and Adjusting Asthma Management

Effective management of pediatric asthma depends on routine visits to the doctor. These meetings enable continual monitoring, changes to the asthma action plan, and discussion of any worries or inquiries.

Components of Regular Check-Ups:

1. **Assessment of Asthma Control:** Healthcare professionals evaluate the child's asthma control, taking into account the frequency and intensity of symptoms, peak flow readings, and medication usage.

2. **Medication Review:** The healthcare professional examines the child's existing medication schedule, evaluates its efficacy, and makes any necessary modifications.

3. **Lung Function Tests:** Spirometry is one type of lung function test that may be used to assess lung function and track changes over time.

4. **Review of Triggers:** The medical professional discusses possible asthma

triggers and provides advice on reducing exposure.

5. **Asthma Education:** Regular checkups offer the chance for asthma education, making sure that the kid and any caregivers are aware of the illness and equipped to handle it.

6. **Asthma Action Plan Updates:** Updates to the child's asthma action plan are produced as appropriate depending on the evaluation and any modifications to asthma management.

Frequency of Check-Ups:

Depending on the child's asthma severity and management, different checkup intervals are recommended. Children with asthma who are well-controlled may need checkups every six to twelve months, while those with asthma who are not as well-controlled may need more regular visits.

A multifaceted strategy is needed to prevent asthma attacks in kids, including reducing triggers, establishing an asthma-friendly home environment, assuring helpful school accommodations, encouraging immunizations, and going to frequent checkups. Parents, caregivers, and healthcare professionals may collaborate to lower the risk of asthma exacerbations and provide children with asthma the chance to live healthy, active lives by focusing on four essential elements of asthma prevention.

Chapter 4

Medications and Treatment Options

In order to effectively control asthma, patients frequently combine prescription drugs with dietary changes and preventative measures. Let's examine the many drugs used to treat asthma, go through proper inhaler and nebulizer techniques, and think about complementary and alternative therapies that might be utilized in addition to standard asthma treatment.

Overview of Asthma Medications

Long-term control medications and quick-relief (rescue) medications are the two basic categories into which asthma medications may be broadly categorized. Each kind has a particular function in the treatment of asthma symptoms.

Long-Term Control Medications

Daily usage of long-term control medications is required to prevent and maintain long-term control of asthma symptoms. They assist in lowering airway inflammation and preventing asthma attacks. Several typical long-term control medications are:

1. **Inhaled Corticosteroids (ICS):** The best - most effective long-term control medications for lowering airway inflammation are inhaled corticosteroids (ICS), which are administered by inhalers or nebulizers. They are typically administered

as the first line of defense against recurrent asthma.

2. **Long-Acting Beta-Agonists (LABA):** LABAs (Long-Acting beta agonists) are bronchodilators that aid in relaxing the muscles of the airways. They are frequently administered in combination with ICS for patients with moderate to severe asthma.

3. **Leukotriene Modifiers:** These medications assist in decreasing inflammation by inhibiting the function of leukotrienes, which are chemicals that contribute to asthma symptoms. They are offered as chewable tablets or pills.

4. **Mast Cell Stabilizers:** These drugs work to stop the release of chemicals that irritate the airways. They are normally given using a

nebulizer and are frequently used in children with moderate asthma.

5. **Biologics:** In some situations, patients with severe asthma are given biologic medications. These medications specifically target elements of the immune system that cause asthma symptoms.

Quick-Relief (Rescue) Medications

When asthma symptoms abruptly intensify or during asthma attacks, quick-relief medications offer immediate relief. They function by loosening the muscles that surround the airways, which facilitates breathing. Typical treatments for immediate relief include:

1. **Short-Acting Beta-Agonists (SABA):** SABAs, like albuterol, are often delivered via

inhalers or nebulizers and offer prompt relief from asthma symptoms.

2. **Ipratropium Bromide:** This drug is used in conjunction with SABAs to relieve severe asthma exacerbations further.

3. **Oral Corticosteroids:** In some circumstances, doctors may prescribe short-term usage of oral corticosteroids to manage severe asthma symptoms.

It's crucial to remember that a healthcare professional should prescribe asthma medications depending on the severity of your child's asthma and their particular requirements. Effective management of asthma requires strict adherence to the prescribed medication regimen.

Inhalers and Nebulizers: How to Use Them Correctly

To administer asthma medications directly to the airways, common delivery methods include inhalers and nebulizers. For the medication to successfully reach the lungs, these devices must be used correctly. Here are some pointers for properly using inhalers and nebulizers:

Using Inhalers (Metered-Dose Inhalers or MDIs):

1. **Shake the Inhaler:** To make sure the medicine is evenly mixed, shake the inhaler thoroughly before each use.

2. **Prime the Inhaler:** Follow the manufacturer's directions to prime the inhaler if it's new or hasn't been used in a while.

3. **Stand Upright:** Hold the inhaler upright with the mouthpiece at the bottom while standing straight.

4. **Breathe Out:** Exhale completely after taking a long breath to clear your lungs.

5. **Seal Your Lips:** Put the mouthpiece in between your lips and seal them around it.

6. **Inhale Slowly:** Start breathing deeply and slowly through the mouthpiece while applying pressure to the canister of the inhaler.

7. **Hold Breath:** After taking a breath, hold it for around 10 seconds to give the medicine time to enter your airways.

8. **Exhale Slowly:** Breathe out gradually and softly.

9. **Wait:** If a second puff is necessary, wait the advised amount of time (often between 30 seconds and one minute) before doing the action again.

10. **Rinse Mouth:** After taking corticosteroid inhalers, rinse your mouth thoroughly with water to lessen the chance of developing oral thrush.

Spacers

Effective Medication Delivery

To administer asthma drugs directly to the airways, inhalers are frequently utilized. However, it may be challenging for young children in particular to use inhalers efficiently. Spacers, commonly referred to as holding chambers, can enhance the administration of medications and facilitate medication inhalation in children.

Advantages of Spacers:

1. **Improved Medication Deposition:** By ensuring that more of the medicine enters the lungs and airways, spacers assist in lessening the risk of adverse effects and boost the treatment's efficiency.

2. **Ease of Use:** Children who have trouble controlling the breathing process with a regular inhaler may find spacers to be very helpful.

3. **Reduced Oral Thrush Risk:** When corticosteroid inhalers are used directly in the mouth, there is a chance of developing oral thrush, a fungal infection.

4. **Adaptability:** Spacers are versatile for use with different types of asthma treatments since they may be used with

both metered-dose inhalers (MDIs) and dry powder inhalers (DPIs).

Using Spacers with Inhalers:

1. Connect the spacer to the inhaler.

2. As instructed, shake the inhaler canister.

3. Tell the child to put the mouthpiece of the spacer in their mouth and create a secure seal with their lips.

4. While the child inhales slowly and deeply, depress the inhaler canister to release the medicine.

5. After a little period of holding your breath, slowly let it out.

6. If taking corticosteroid inhalers, rinse the child's mouth thoroughly with water to reduce the possibility of oral thrush.

Cleaning and Maintenance:

To avoid the accumulation of drug residue, spacers should be cleaned often in accordance with the manufacturer's recommendations.

Using Nebulizers:

1. **Wash Hands:** Start by properly washing your hands to maintain cleanliness.

2. **Assemble the Nebulizer:** Assemble the nebulizer in accordance with the directions provided by the manufacturer.

3. **Measure Medication:** Use a clean, dry syringe to measure the recommended dosage of medication.

4. **Place Medication:** Fill the medicine cup in the nebulizer with the measured medication.

5. **Connect Tubing:** Connect the tubing to the air compressor and nebulizer.

6. **Attach Mouthpiece or Mask:** Join the nebulizer's mouthpiece or mask.

7. **Turn on Compressor:** Start the air compressor and check to see if the mouthpiece or mask is emitting a steady mist.

8. Breathe Normally: Encourage your child to inhale and exhale normally through the mouthpiece or mask.

9. **Continue Until Empty:** The Nebulization process should be continued until the drug cup is empty, which typically takes 10 to 15 minutes.

10. **Turn Off the Compressor:** Switch off the air compressor, remove the tubing, and

disassemble the nebulizer so that it may be cleaned.

In order to guarantee proper inhaler and nebulizer technique, both parents and kids must get the necessary instruction from a healthcare professional or asthma educator. Visits to medical professionals on a regular basis can also assist in evaluating and enhancing the usage of nebulizers and inhalers.

Alternative and Complementary Therapies

Some parents look towards complementary and alternative therapies in addition to traditional asthma drugs to help control the condition. Before including these therapies in your child's asthma treatment plan, it's crucial to proceed with caution and speak with a healthcare professional. Some complementary and alternative therapies investigated for the treatment of asthma include:

1. **Breathing Exercises:** Exercises that enhance lung function and lessen symptoms include diaphragmatic breathing and pursed-lip breathing.

2. **Acupuncture:** Although there is little scientific proof - evidence, several asthmatics have found relief from acupuncture sessions.

3. **Yoga:** Through regulated breathing methods and moderate activities, yoga can boost lung function and induce relaxation.

4. **Herbal Remedies:** A number of plants, including ginger and licorice root, have

been investigated for their possible ability to reduce inflammation in the airways.

5. **Dietary Modifications:** Changing one's diet to include more fruits, vegetables, and omega-3 fatty acids may help reduce the symptoms of asthma.

6. **Mind-Body Therapies:** Techniques like mindfulness and meditation can help you manage stress, which can exacerbate the symptoms of asthma.

While some people may find relief from complementary and alternative therapies, it's important to keep in mind that they should never be used in place of prescription asthma medications. Before introducing any alternative therapies into your child's asthma control strategy, always check with their doctor.

The creation of an asthma action plan, lifestyle and nutritional issues, and methods for controlling asthma at work and in social situations will all be covered as we go along. With this information, you will be well-equipped to successfully manage the challenges of controlling your child's asthma.

Chapter 5

Developing an Asthma Action Plan

A peak flow or asthma action plan, also known as an asthma diary, is a vital tool for accurately identifying and treating your child's asthma. It supports the tracking of symptoms, triggering events, medication use, and peak flow measurements over time by parents, caregivers, and healthcare providers. With the assistance of this tailored plan, you and your kid may confidently face the challenges of asthma. It specifies the actions to take in various scenarios. Let's now examine the function of an asthma action plan, walk you through developing a personal plan with your doctor, and give you crucial advice on what to do while having an asthma attack.

The Role of an Asthma Action Plan in Managing the Condition

An asthma action plan is a written guide that details how to take care of your child's asthma. It is intended to assist you, your kid, and anybody else responsible for their care in understanding what to do in various circumstances, from managing your child's asthma on a regular basis to dealing with asthma exacerbations. An asthma action plan is necessary for the following reasons:

1. **Objective Data:** An asthma diary offers objective data that can help medical professionals make precise diagnoses and therapy changes - treatment adjustments.

2.   **Pattern   Recognition:**   Observing symptoms and triggers over time might assist in seeing patterns or trends that aren't always obvious during treatment visits.

3. **Personalized Guidance:** An asthma action plan is made specifically for your child's symptoms,   triggers,   and   prescription medications.   It   offers   individualized guidance tailored to your child's particular requirements.

4. **Clear Communication:** It acts as a tool for communication between you, your kid, healthcare professionals, educators, and caretakers. Everyone is likely to be on the same page about the management of asthma when there is a consistent strategy in place.

5. **Day-to-day Management:** A written asthma action plan can be used to monitor your daily asthma management, such as peak flow measurements and medication regimens. It makes sure that asthma medications are taken regularly and according to instructions.

6. **Asthma Exacerbation Response:** In the case of an asthma attack or exacerbation, the action plan describes what to do to offer immediate relief and when to seek medical attention.

7. **Empowerment:** A written asthma action plan gives your kid the ability to actively participate in their asthma management. It gives them a feeling of control and assurance when managing their illness.

Creating a Customized Plan with Your Healthcare Provider

Your kid, your healthcare practitioner, and you will work together to create a unique asthma action plan. It's important to include your child in this process as they become older since it makes them more accountable for managing their asthma. The following are the essential elements of an asthma action plan:

1. **Personal Information:** Provide the name, birthdate, emergency phone numbers, and contact information for the healthcare professional.

2. **Asthma Severity Classification:** Based on your child's symptoms, medication use, and lung function, your doctor will determine how severe your child's asthma is. The

treatment strategy is guided by this categorization.

3. **Medication Instructions:** Indicate the names of your child's prescription medications, their doses, and the times that they should be taken. Include both short-term medications and long-term control medications. By doing this, medication compliance is improved.

4. **Peak Flow Zones:** Using a peak flow meter, you may assess how well your kid can breathe in and out. Based on your child's individual best peak flow measurement, your healthcare professional will develop peak flow zones (green, yellow, and red). These zones show how well asthma is controlled.

Dr. George K. Shelley

- **Green Zone:** Asthma is under good control in this area. Asthma symptoms are stable, therefore your kid should keep taking the recommended daily controller drugs.

- **Yellow Zone:** This zone signals caution. It indicates that the asthma your kid has is getting worse, and action has to be taken to treat this. Usually, this entails temporarily raising the dosage of the controlling drug.

- **Red Zone:** A serious asthma attack or exacerbation is indicated by the red zone. In order to treat the symptoms, quick-relief medications and seeking medical attention may both need to be used.

91

5. **Asthma Triggers:** Identify prevalent asthma triggers for your child and discuss ways to prevent or limit exposure to these triggers.

6. **Asthma Symptoms:** Describe the common symptoms your kid encounters when their asthma flares up. This makes it easier for you and your kid to spot when their asthma is getting worse.

7. **Emergency Contacts:** Include a list of emergency contacts that includes the phone numbers for your child's doctor, the neighborhood hospital, and any specialists who are engaged in their treatment.

8. **Instructions for What to Do:** Based on the peak flow zone, provide precise, step-by-step guidance on what to do while experiencing an asthma attack:

- In the **Green Zone,** Take your daily controller medications as directed.

- In the **Yellow Zone**, abide by your healthcare provider's detailed recommendations for modifying medication dose.

- In the **Red Zone**, start emergency procedures, such as utilizing quick-relief medications, and seek emergency medical assistance.

9. **Peak Flow Readings:** If the asthma care plan includes peak flow monitoring, take regular peak flow measurements. This sheds light on how lung function varies.

Whether at home, school or when traveling, keep a copy of your child's asthma action plan on hand at all times. Make sure that the plan is communicated to the teachers, caregivers, and school staff.

Chapter 6

When to Seek Emergency Care

With the right care and assistance, childhood asthma may typically be effectively treated. The need to know when to seek emergency treatment and to be ready for the likelihood of severe asthma attacks cannot be overstated. Here, we'll look at how to spot severe asthma attacks, what to do in an emergency situation involving asthma, going to the hospital, comprehending the long-term effects of having uncontrolled asthma, and being ready for crises.

Recognizing Severe Asthma Attacks

Identifying Signs of a Severe Asthma Attack

Many asthmatic kids have mild to moderate symptoms that may be controlled at home, but some could have severe asthma attacks that need to be treated right away by a doctor. For prompt intervention, it is essential to recognize the warning indications of a severe asthma attack.

Common Signs of a Severe Asthma Attack:

1. **Extreme Breathlessness:** The child may have difficulty speaking or may take short, shallow breaths.

2. **Severe Wheezing:** During both intake and exhale, wheezing is loud and noticeable.

3. **Coughing:** Severe, persistent cough that does not go better with treatment.

4. **Cyanosis:** The child may have blue or gray lips, skin, or nails as a result of oxygen deprivation.

5. **Inability to Lie Down:** In order to breathe comfortably, the child may need to sit up or lean forward.

6. **Use of Accessory Muscles:** The child may be able to breathe more easily by using his or her neck and chest muscles.

7. **No Improvement with Rescue Inhaler:** Using a rescue inhaler does not bring about immediate relief.

What to Do During an Asthma Emergency:

When a kid is experiencing a severe asthma attack, it's critical to respond quickly and appropriately to protect their safety and well-being. Even though an asthma attack might be terrifying, you can respond appropriately if you have an asthma action plan in place. The general procedures to follow during an asthma attack are as follows:

Steps to Take During an Asthma Emergency:

1. **Stay Calm:** Try to maintain your composure while reassuring the child. Panic and anxiety may make things worse.

2. **Administer Rescue Inhaler:** If the kid has a rescue inhaler that was prescribed, use it as instructed. Provide four puffs using a

spacer (or as prescribed per their asthma action plan).

3. **Call 911 or Emergency Services:** If after taking the rescue inhaler the child's symptoms do not improve or if they get worse, call 911 or emergency services right away.

4. **Continue to Administer Medication:** If the child's breathing is still difficult after 20 minutes, continue giving the rescue inhaler every 20 minutes (up to three doses) while you wait for emergency assistance.

5. **Monitor the Child:** Keep a watchful check on the child's breathing, heartbeat, and skin tone. If the child stops breathing and has no pulse, be ready to administer CPR.

6. **Review and Adjust:** After an asthma episode, talk with your doctor about what

could have caused it in order to identify any potential triggers or changes that should be made to the action plan.

Keep in mind that asthma attacks can range in intensity, and that prompt treatment is essential to avoiding a more serious episode. With the help of your child's doctor, review and update your child's asthma action plan on a regular basis to make sure it still applies to their current situation.

Visiting the Emergency Room: When Emergency Room Care is Necessary

In some circumstances, severe asthma attacks may need a trip to the emergency department in order to receive prompt medical attention.

When to Go to the Emergency Room:

1. **Severe Symptoms Persist:** When a child's symptoms are severe even after taking the rescue inhaler as instructed, it is crucial to seek emergency treatment.

2. **Difficulty Speaking:** If the youngster has trouble speaking or is unable to talk because they are out of breath, this is a symptom of extreme discomfort.

3. **Use of Accessory Muscles:** Severe respiratory distress is indicated if the child's neck and chest muscles are clearly straining hard to breathe.

4. **Cyanosis:** The child needs emergency medical care right away if their lips, face, or nails turn blue or gray as a result of oxygen deprivation.

5. Drowsiness or Altered Mental State: A child who starts to feel drowsy, disoriented, or shows changes in their level of mental awareness needs to be evaluated right away.

6. Ineffective Medication: Do not wait to seek emergency treatment if the kid does not respond to the rescue inhaler or if their health deteriorates.

Long-Term Consequences of Uncontrolled Asthma

The Importance of Timely Intervention

Lack of asthma control and management can have long-term effects on a child's respiratory health and general well-being. This is especially true during severe attacks.

Potential Long-Term Consequences:

1. **Reduced Lung Function:** Uncontrolled asthma can cause persistent inflammation and airway remodeling, which over time can lead to diminished lung function.

2. **Frequent Hospitalizations:** Serious asthma attacks that need hospitalization might interfere with a child's daily activities and schooling.

3. **Emotional Impact:** Children who experience frequent asthma flare-ups and ER visits may experience mental distress, anxiety, and fear.

4. **Missed School and Activities:** Asthma that is not under control can cause missed classes as well as reduced involvement in social and physical activities.

5. **Financial Costs:** The cost of hospital stays and ER visits can put a strain on families.

Staying Prepared for Emergencies

Effective management of childhood asthma crises depends on preparation. Families and caregivers should take precautions to be ready for asthma emergencies.

Key Preparedness Measures:

1. **Asthma Action Plan:** Ensure that the child has an up-to-date asthma action plan, and routinely go through it with the child's healthcare professionals.

2. **Emergency Contacts:** Maintain a list of emergency contacts, including doctors, the child's school, and the neighborhood emergency services.

3. **Medication Accessibility:** Maintain easy access to your asthma meds and make sure your family and caregivers are aware of their location.

4. **Rescue Inhaler and Spacer:** When you're not at home, always have a rescue inhaler and spacer with you.

5. **Asthma Diary:** Keep an asthma journal to keep note of your symptoms, triggers, and medication usage. This can help you spot patterns and will provide you with important information in an emergency.

6. **Emergency Kit:** Consider putting together an emergency pack for your child's asthma that contains their meds, a peak flow meter, a spacer, a copy of the action plan, and emergency contact information.

7. **Education:** Inform teachers, family members, and other support people about the child's asthma action plan and how to act in an emergency.

8. **Regular Follow-Up:** Keep setting up routine follow-up meetings with medical professionals to evaluate your asthma control and make any required modifications to your treatment plan.

Essential components of managing childhood asthma include identifying the warning signs of severe asthma attacks, acting appropriately during an asthma emergency, knowing when to go to the emergency room, comprehending the potential long-term effects of uncontrolled asthma, and being ready for emergencies. Parents, caregivers, and healthcare professionals may collaborate to safeguard the safety and well-being of children with asthma and lessen the negative effects of severe asthma attacks on their lives by being knowledgeable and proactive.

After that, you should think about your child's food and way of life, as well as how to manage it at school and in social situations. You should also take proactive measures to make your child's surroundings asthma-friendly.

Chapter 7

Lifestyle and Diet for Asthma Management

Management of asthma goes beyond prescription medications and medical attention. Dietary and lifestyle choices are very important for managing asthma symptoms and enhancing your child's general health. A healthy lifestyle involves things like proper eating, exercise, rest, and stress reduction. Let's examine the relationship between diet and nutrition and asthma, consider physical activity for children with asthma, and discuss stress management strategies to improve your child's asthma management strategy.

The Impact of Diet and Nutrition on Asthma

Diet and nutrition can alter asthma symptoms in addition to having a direct impact on general health. Even while asthma cannot be cured by food alone, several dietary options and nutrients may help control symptoms and lower the likelihood of exacerbations. Here are some dietary recommendations for managing asthma:

1. **Anti-Inflammatory Foods:** Including anti-inflammatory foods in your child's diet may help lessen the inflammation of the airways that comes with asthma. Fruits, vegetables, whole grains, nuts, and seeds are some examples of these foods. Omega-3 fatty acids, which are also included in flaxseeds

and fatty seafood like salmon, have anti-inflammatory qualities.

2. **Vitamin D:** Having enough vitamin D levels may help to lessen the symptoms of asthma. Encourage your child to spend time outside and think about vitamin D-enriched meals such as fortified milk or orange juice. Before beginning any supplements, speak with your child's doctor.

3. **Antioxidants:** Antioxidants, such as vitamins C and E, can aid in preventing inflammation of the airways. Vitamin C may be found in citrus fruits, berries, and nuts, whereas vitamin E can be found in seeds, nuts, and vegetable oils.

4. **Magnesium:** According to some research, foods high in magnesium, such as leafy greens, nuts, and whole grains, may aid in

relaxing the airways and have a bronchodilator impact.

5. **Hydration:** For those who have asthma, maintaining proper hydration is crucial. As dehydration can thicken mucus and exacerbate asthma symptoms, maintaining enough hydration helps keep airway secretions thin and encourages better breathing.

6. **Avoiding Trigger Foods:** Some people's asthma symptoms may be worse by certain meals. Dairy products, eggs, and processed foods with plenty of preservatives and chemicals are common trigger foods. Be aware of your child's food triggers and talk to your doctor about them.

7. **Maintaining a Healthy Weight:** Asthma symptoms might get worse with obesity. To

help your child keep a healthy weight, promote a balanced diet and frequent exercise.

8. **Allergen Management:** Allergen management is essential if your kid suffers from both asthma and food allergies. Doing so will help to avoid allergic responses that could aggravate asthma symptoms.

9. **Dietary Restrictions:** Consult a trained dietitian or other healthcare professional if your kid has unique dietary needs or allergies to make sure they get the nourishment they need without exacerbating their asthma symptoms.

10. **Balanced Diet:** A healthy diet should contain plenty of fruits, vegetables, whole grains, lean proteins, and dairy products. Encourage your child to follow this advice. A

healthy diet can promote overall well-being and perhaps lessen asthma symptoms.

Before making large dietary alterations, it is important to speak with your child's healthcare physician or a certified dietitian because individual reactions to dietary changes might differ.

Exercise and Physical Activity for Kids with Asthma

Even for kids with asthma, exercise is a crucial component of a healthy lifestyle. Regular exercise helps strengthen respiratory muscles, improve lung function, increase self-confidence, and improve general fitness. How to promote exercise and physical activity in children with asthma is as follows:

1. **Consult with Healthcare Provider:** Consult your child's healthcare physician before beginning or making changes to an exercise program to verify that it is secure and suitable for the severity and control of your child's asthma.

2. **Choose Asthma-Friendly Activities:** Some sports and exercises have a lower risk of bringing on asthma symptoms. For instance, swimming is frequently accepted well because the warm, muggy air surrounding the pool can be calming to the airways. Exercises like riding, yoga, and walking are also appropriate.

3. **Use Pre-Exercise Medications:** Applying a quick-relief drug (such as albuterol) prior to exercise can help avoid exercise-induced bronchoconstriction (EIB) if advised to do so by your child's doctor.

4. **Warm-Up and Cool Down:** Encourage your child to warm up before activity and cool down afterward at all times. This lowers the likelihood of asthma symptoms while helping the body get ready for exercise.

5. **Monitor Symptoms:** Teaching your child to be aware of their asthma symptoms while exercising will help you to monitor symptoms. They should cease participating in the activity and follow the instructions on their quick-relief prescription medication if they start coughing, wheezing, having trouble breathing, or feeling their chest tighten.

6. **Asthma-Friendly Sports:** Encourage your kid to take part in sports that are asthma-friendly. In activities like track and field,

cross-country running, and martial arts, many kids with asthma do quite well.

7. **Asthma Action Plan:** Make sure that the asthma action plan for your kid addresses how to control the condition while engaging in physical activity. Coaches, physical education instructors, and other caregivers should be made aware of this strategy.

8. **Promote Enjoyment:** Stress the value of having fun while exercising. Children are more likely to continue being active when they find an activity they enjoy.

9. **Gradual Progression:** Encourage moderate increases in physical activity. Start with briefer, less strenuous workouts, then progressively increase both duration and intensity.

10. **Consider Individual Preferences:** When choosing activities, take the child's interests and preferences into consideration. If kids are having fun while exercising, they are more likely to keep moving – and stay active.

Exercise-Induced Bronchoconstriction (EIB):

Children suffering from asthma may have exercise-induced bronchoconstriction (EIB), a condition in which physical activity triggers asthma symptoms. To manage EIB:

- Before a workout, take the bronchodilators as advised.

- Make sure your workout plan includes a warm-up and cool-down.

- Take into account activities that need brief bursts of effort, like martial arts.

Communication with Coaches and Teachers:

The child's asthma should be brought up with coaches, physical education teachers, and activity leaders. Make sure they are aware of any special accommodations or instructions by going over the asthma action plan with them.

Stress Management Techniques

Some people's asthma symptoms might get worse under stress. Teaching your kid stress management methods can be an important component of their asthma management strategy. The following strategies for handling stress are appropriate for kids:

1. **Deep Breathing:** Encourage your kids to use deep breathing techniques to unwind and calm their minds. Deeply inhale

through the nose, hold for a moment, and then slowly exhale through the mouth.

2. **Yoga and Mindfulness:** Exercises like yoga and mindfulness training can lower stress and enhance mental health. If possible, let your kid attend classes or practice at home with internet tools.

3. **Regular Relaxation:** Include routine relaxation time in your child's schedule, either before bed or during stressful periods. Use methods like guided imagery or progressive muscular relaxation.

4. **Open Communication:** Open communication is something you should encourage with your kids. Encourage them to communicate their emotions and worries while listening sympathetically.

5. **Create a Calm Environment:** Establish a Calm Environment: Make sure that your child's home is a calm one. Reduce your exposure to stresses like long screen times and loud places.

6. **Time Management:** Teach your child time management techniques to lessen the stress brought on by deadlines and scheduling.

7. **Healthy Lifestyle Habits:** Promote a balanced lifestyle that includes enough sleep, frequent exercise, and good food to help manage stress.

8. **Adequate Sleep:** Getting enough sleep is important for children with asthma. Maintaining a regular sleep pattern and getting enough rest can help avoid fatigue, which can make asthma symptoms worse.

9. **Seek Professional Help:** If your child consistently feels stressed out or is having emotional problems, consult a therapist or counselor.

You may aid your kid in managing stressors that could lead to asthma exacerbations by introducing stress management strategies into their daily routine.

The next section will discuss how to manage asthma at home, in social situations, and at school. With this information, you will be well-equipped to offer your kid complete assistance for the treatment of their asthma.

Chapter 8

School and Social Life

Managing your child's asthma at school and in social settings is essential for maintaining his or her safety, well-being, and overall quality of life. It's time to look at methods for properly managing asthma at school, educating classmates and teachers, and encouraging your kids to actively participate in their asthma care.

Navigating Asthma at School

Since school plays a key role in a child's life, it's crucial to make sure your child's asthma treatment includes the school setting. Asthma management tips for your child at school include the following:

1. **Create an Asthma Action Plan for School:** Create an asthma action plan specifically for the school setting by working with your child's healthcare practitioner. The severity of your child's asthma, dosage instructions, peak flow zones, and emergency procedures should all be covered in this plan.

2. **Meet with School Staff:** Arrange a meeting with your child's teachers, school nurse, and other pertinent school personnel to go over the asthma action plan. Make sure that everyone is aware of their responsibility for helping control your child's asthma.

3. **Provide Necessary Medications:** Ensure the school has a sufficient amount of your child's prescription asthma medications, especially quick-relief inhalers. Provide

Necessary Medications. Your child should be aware of where these drugs are kept and that they should be easily accessible.

4. **Educate School Personnel:** Educate teachers, coaches, and other members of the school staff about asthma, including symptoms, causes, and emergency measures. Offer teaching on how to make use of your child's inhaler or nebulizer if necessary.

5. **Asthma-Friendly Classroom:** Advocate for an asthma-friendly classroom by asking for modifications like air purifiers, efforts to reduce allergens, and attention to your child's asthma triggers.

6. **Lunch and Allergen Considerations:** If your kid suffers from both asthma and food allergies, let the school cafeteria staff know

so that they may make sure allergen-free lunch alternatives are available. Ensure that your child is aware of the foods to avoid.

7. **Physical Education and Sports:** Talk to the coaches and physical education instructor about your child's asthma. Make sure your kid has access to their quick-relief prescription while engaging in physical activity, and provide instructions for managing symptoms brought on by exercise.

8. **Field Trips and Extracurricular Activities:** Before field trips and extracurricular activities, let the school administration know your kid has asthma. Make sure your child has access to their asthma action plan and medicines on these occasions.

Educating Teachers and Classmates

A caring and understanding atmosphere for your kid may be created by educating teachers and classmates about asthma. How to approach asthma education is as follows:

1. **Teacher Training:** At the start of each school year or whenever a new teacher takes over, ask for a quick asthma education session for your child's teacher(s). Give them written information on your child's unique needs, as well as information about asthma.

2. **Classroom Presentation:** If your child is at ease with it, think about setting up a little presentation about asthma in the school. Your kid can describe their illness, show

how they use an inhaler, and offer advice on how peers can be helpful.

3. **Asthma Education Materials:** Provide age-appropriate asthma education resources to the school for distribution to instructors and students, such as books or pamphlets.

4. **Open Communication:** Encourage instructors and classmates to ask questions and voice their worries about your child's asthma through open communication. Clear communication helps clear up misunderstandings and fosters a positive environment.

5. **Bullying Prevention:** Discuss how crucial it is to stop bullying of people with asthma. Encourage your child to report any bullying incidents to the school authorities and

teach them coping mechanisms for handling possible bullying scenarios.

6. **Inclusion and Support:** Encourage teachers to involve your child in every activity in the classroom, which includes physical education and group projects. Most children with asthma may engage completely in school activities with the right asthma management.

Encouraging Independence and Self-Care

As your kid matures, it's crucial to encourage independence and the development of self-care abilities linked to managing asthma. Here's how to motivate your kid to actively participate in their asthma treatment:

1. **Age-Appropriate Responsibility:** Assign your kid asthma management tasks that are in line with their age. While older children can learn to take responsibility for their medicine and adhere to their asthma action plan, younger children may require more supervision.

2. **Medication Self-Administration:** Teach your child how to regularly and correctly use his or her nebulizer, spacer, and inhaler. Allowing children to take medication of their own with supervision should be gradually introduced. As children get older, encourage them to manage their medication routine on their own.

3. **Peak Flow Monitoring:** If necessary, show your kid how to check their lung function using a peak flow meter. Teach them to identify peak flow zones and to

take appropriate action in accordance with their asthma action plan.

4. **Emergency Response:** Make sure your kid is aware of the appropriate actions to take in the event of an asthma attack, including when and how to use their rescue inhaler or other quick-relief medicine.

5. **Asthma Diary:** Encourage your kid to keep an asthma diary or notebook to keep track of their symptoms, allergen triggers, and medication usage. They may be able to comprehend their asthma patterns better as a result of this.

6. **Self-Advocacy:** Teach your child to speak out for their own needs related to their asthma. This includes being able to express their requirements to peers, instructors,

and other people as well as understanding when to ask for assistance.

7. **Supportive Environment:** Establish a setting where your child is at ease talking about their asthma and asking questions. Be a source of inspiration and assistance.

8. **Symptom Recognition:** Teach kids to recognize asthma symptoms and the need for early intervention when symptoms worsen.

9. **Lifestyle Choices:** Encourage kids to have healthy lifestyles by modeling behaviors like eating a balanced diet, exercising regularly, and abstaining from smoking or being around those who are smoking.

Gradual Independence: As children mature, gradually hand over duties to them in order to foster self-management abilities.

You are giving your kid the tools they need to properly manage their asthma as they enter adolescence and adulthood by encouraging independence and self-care abilities.

Chapter 9

Support for Parents and Caregivers

It can be difficult to provide both practical and emotional support for a kid who has asthma. As a responsible parent or caregiver, you play an important part in your child's asthma management. Here, we'll look at coping mechanisms, support systems, and the significance of self-care for caregivers as they work through emotional and practical challenges.

The Emotional Impact of Asthma

Children and their families may experience emotional and psychological effects from childhood asthma. For thorough asthma management, it is essential to comprehend and address these emotional aspects.

Common Emotional Responses:

1. **Anxiety:** Asthmatic children may suffer anxiety as a result of asthma attacks or the fear of being unable to breathe.

2. **Frustration:** Children may find it difficult to deal with the restrictions that asthma might impose, such as skipping school or social events.

3. **Depression:** Long-term management of a chronic illness, such as asthma, can cause depressive symptoms, particularly if it interferes with a child's day-to-day activities.

4. **Stigma:** Children with asthma may experience stigma because of

misunderstandings or a lack of knowledge about the condition among peers.

Coping with the Emotional Challenges

A wide range of emotions can be experienced when raising an asthmatic child. Experiences of fear, worry, frustration, and even guilt are completely normal. Managing these feelings is crucial to giving your child the best care possible. The following are some tactics for handling emotional difficulties:

1. **Education and Awareness:** To better understand the condition, educate yourself, your child, and everyone else in the home about asthma, its management, and the significance of adhering to treatment. When you are well-informed, you can feel more in control, which reduces anxiety.

2. **Open Communication:** Maintain open lines of communication with your child regarding their asthma. Reassure them that you are there to support them and encourage them to express their feelings and worries.

3. **Seek Support:** Don't be afraid to ask for help from healthcare professionals who have experience with chronic illness and can offer advice on how to manage emotions, such as therapists or counselors.

4. **Support Groups:** Joining a support group for parents of children with asthma is something you might want to do. Making connections with people who have gone through similar things can be reassuring and insightful.

5. **Self-Care:** Set maintaining your physical and emotional well-being as a top priority. You can better care for your child if you take care of yourself.

6. **Resilience Building:** Building resilience involves using mindfulness, stress-reduction techniques, and positive thinking. These abilities can aid you in overcoming obstacles more successfully.

7. **Celebrate Achievements:** Honor the accomplishments and landmarks your child has made in managing their asthma. Their confidence and motivation can both be increased by positive reinforcement.

Coping with the Practical Challenges

The management of your child's asthma may present practical difficulties, such as managing medication schedules, scheduling doctor visits, and creating asthma-friendly environments. Here are some useful tactics to assist you in overcoming these difficulties:

1. **Asthma Action Plan:** Carefully adhere to the asthma action plan that your child's doctor has provided. This strategy provides a road map for successfully managing asthma.

2. **Medication Management:** Establish a system for managing medications, such as by setting up pillboxes or inhaler reminders. To ensure you never run out of medication, keep track of all refills.

3. **Healthcare Appointments:** Keep a calendar or digital scheduler handy to keep

track of your doctor's appointments, prescription refills, and asthma checkups.

4. **Asthma-Friendly Home:** Reduce allergens and irritants to create an asthma-friendly environment in your home. Use allergen-proof bedding covers, do regular cleaning and vacuuming, and keep the right humidity levels.

5. **Emergency Preparedness:** Prepare an emergency kit with your child's medications for their asthma, a copy of their asthma action plan, and crucial contact information. Make sure you and your child are both aware of where the kit is.

6. **School Coordination:** Maintain regular contact with your child's school to make sure they have a welcoming and secure environment for managing their asthma.

7. **Flexibility:** Be ready for unanticipated asthma flare-ups. It is essential to have a backup childcare strategy and to know when to seek medical help.

Building a Support Network

Your ability to manage the difficulties of raising an asthmatic child will be greatly impacted by the strength of your support system. How to create a support system is as follows:

1. **Family and Friends:** Contact your family and friends, who can offer you emotional support and help with childcare if necessary.

Make sure that the child's siblings and other caregivers are aware of his or her asthma action plan and are prepared to help if necessary.

Establish a welcoming environment where the child can talk about their asthma and express their emotions.

Recognize the child's efforts in asthma management and offer encouragement and supportive feedback.

2. **Healthcare Team:** Build a close bond with your child's medical team, which should include pediatricians, asthma specialists, nurses, and therapists. They can provide direction and assurance.

3. **Peer Support:** Introduce asthmatic kids to local groups or online forums where they can communicate with other kids going through similar experiences. Sharing experiences can be both comforting and instructive.

4. **Support Groups:** Join a support group for parents of asthmatic kids in your area or online. These groups can offer insightful knowledge, compassion, and comprehension.

5. **School Community:** Join the school community by talking to the other parents, teachers, and nurses there. The management of your child's asthma can be improved through cooperation with the school.

6. **Therapist or Counselor:** If emotional difficulties become overwhelming, think about consulting a therapist or counselor for yourself or your child.

7. **Parenting Classes:** Attend parenting workshops or classes that concentrate on managing children's chronic illnesses. These

can offer helpful coping mechanisms and strategies.

Self-Care for Caregivers

Self-care is not selfish; it is a crucial component of giving your child the best care possible. The following are self-care techniques for caregivers:

1. **Prioritize Sleep:** You need restorative sleep in order to maintain your physical and emotional well-being.

2. **Healthy Eating:** Maintain your energy and health by eating a balanced diet. Your resilience may be increased by proper nutrition.

3. **Exercise:** Take part in regular physical activity to keep your body healthy overall and reduce stress.

4. **Me-Time:** Schedule time just for you, whether it be for relaxation exercises, hobbies, or reading. This replenishes your emotional energy.

5. **Delegate Responsibilities:** Don't be afraid to ask for assistance and assign duties as needed. You do not have an obligation to work alone.

6. **Set Boundaries:** Create limits to avoid burnout. Prioritize your well-being and understand when to say "no."

7. **Professional Support:** If you're having trouble with stress, anxiety, or depression, get professional help. Counselors or therapists can offer insightful guidance.

Keep in mind that by caring for yourself, you can provide better care for your child. You will be better able to manage the difficulties of raising an asthmatic child and give them the love and support they require if you put self-care first.

Chapter 10

Thriving with Asthma

Many kids with asthma not only successfully manage their condition but also excel in many other areas of their lives. Asthma is a medical condition that can be managed. Let's discuss the significance of creating goals and ambitions for kids with asthma, share heartwarming success stories of young people who have accepted their asthma, and promote a positive outlook.

Success Stories of Kids Managing Asthma Effectively

Success stories are a great source of motivation and evidence that kids with asthma may have happy, successful lives. Here are a few examples of children who successfully controlled their asthma in real life:

1. **Jessica's Journey to Becoming a Swimmer:** Jessica was diagnosed with asthma when she was a little child, but she didn't allow it to stop her from living a full life. She learned to control her asthma with correct medication use and frequent exercise with the help of her parents and medical team. Jessica continued to swim, which enhanced her lung capacity. She is currently a competitive swimmer, and because of her hard work, she has obtained several medals and scholarships.

2. **Alex's Musical Pursuit:** Playing the trumpet was Alex's passion, but he struggled because of his asthma. He developed the ability to regulate his breathing while playing music under the

direction of his asthma action plan and a committed music instructor. Alex is a skilled trumpet player now, and he even plays in the marching band at his school.

3. **Emily's Artistic Achievement:** Emily fell in love with art when she was a young child. When she participated in creative activities, her parents and teachers saw that her asthma symptoms improved. Emily turned her passion for painting into accolades for her work at the local and provincial levels. Her artistic endeavors give her a platform for self-expression and stress reduction.

4. **Tom's Athletic Excellence:** Despite being diagnosed with asthma, Tom was motivated to thrive in athletics. He pursued track and field with good medication management and discussions with his coach. His dedication paid off, as he won the 400-

meter state championship, demonstrating that asthma need not be a barrier to sports success.

More Examples of Success Stories:

1. **Olympic Athletes:** A number of Olympians, like Jackie Joyner-Kersee and Michael Phelps, have excelled in their sports while having asthma. Their testimonies encourage young asthmatic athletes to achieve their goals.

2. **Advocates and Role Models:** People with asthma who become leaders and role models in their communities help spread awareness and offer support to those going through similar difficulties.

3. **Medical Breakthroughs:** Success stories also include advancements in medical therapies and procedures that have greatly

raised the standard of living for young people with asthma.

4. **Educational Achievements:** Many asthmatic kids have excelled in their academic studies, proving that asthma need not restrict a child's potential.

These stories show that a child's potential is not limited by having asthma. Children are capable of pursuing their interests and achieving their objectives with the correct encouragement, medication control, and a positive outlook.

Encouraging a Positive Mindset

Children with asthma may interpret and handle their disorder quite differently if their perspective is positive. What can be done to promote a good outlook?

1. **Focus on Abilities, Not Limitations:** Encourage your child to think about their abilities rather than their limitations. Encourage them to discover their passions and skills.

2. **Normalize Asthma:** Tell your child that having asthma is a common ailment that a lot of people successfully manage. By telling tales of other asthmatic kids who have accomplished amazing things, you may help them understand and accept their situation.

3. **Open Communication:** Encourage your child to talk to you freely about their asthma. Encourage them to express their emotions, worries, and goals. Actively listen while providing consolation.

4. **Celebrate Achievements:** Honor your child's accomplishments, no matter how

large or small. Applaud their efforts in pursuing their hobbies and controlling their asthma.

5. **Empower Self-Advocacy:** Encourage your child to speak out for their needs related to their asthma. Encourage them to discuss their illness and any required accommodations with their instructors, coaches, and friends.

6. Building Resilience: Teach your child ways to manage stress, problem-solve, and recover from failures to help them build resilience.

7. **Role Models:** Introduce your child to role models, such as sportsmen, artists, or professionals, who have effectively managed their asthma. It might be

motivational to know that others have overcome comparable difficulties.

Setting Goals and Aspirations

A child's ability to set goals and objectives is essential to their growth, and asthma shouldn't stand in the way of those goals. Here's how to support your kid in setting and achieving goals:

1. **Identify Interests:** Encourage your kid to investigate their hobbies and areas of interest by identifying them. Find out what they like doing and what objectives they want to achieve by asking them.

2. **SMART Goals:** Teach your youngster how to develop SMART goals, which stand for "Specific, Measurable, Achievable, Relevant, Time-bound" objectives. Help them divide

their goals into more manageable, smaller steps.

3. **Asthma-Friendly Accommodations:** Make sure your child's objectives take into consideration their asthma with the help of asthma-friendly accommodations. Talk about any changes or accommodations that are required in order for them to safely pursue their goals.

4. **Support and Resources:** Give your child the assistance and materials they require to succeed. This can entail giving them access to lessons, tools, or chances to improve their abilities.

5. **Track Progress:** Encourage your child to keep track of their advancement toward their objectives. Celebrate progress along the road to keep yourself motivated.

6. **Adjust as Needed:** Recognize that objectives may occasionally need to be modified owing to difficulties connected to asthma. Assist your child in staying flexible and adaptable.

7. **Dream Big:** Encourage your child to have high dreams and to have faith in their abilities. Remind them that their ability to breathe is not defined by their asthma; it is simply one aspect of who they are.

8. **Be a Supportive Guide:** Support your kid as they work toward their objectives by being a supportive guide. Offer unwavering love, guidance, and encouragement.

You may empower your kid to flourish with asthma and develop resilience that will benefit them for the rest of their life by encouraging a positive outlook and assisting them in setting and achieving their ambitions.

Chapter 11

The Future of Childhood Asthma

Research and therapy for asthma have advanced significantly, providing promise for better management and a future with fewer instances of asthma. Here, we examine recent developments in the study and management of asthma and talk about the potential for a future with a lower frequency of the disease.

Advances in Asthma Research and Treatment

The study of asthma is a discipline that is always changing, resulting in new discoveries and methods of therapy. Here are some current developments in the study and management of asthma:

1.   **Biological   Therapies:**   Biologics, commonly referred to as biological treatments, have completely changed how asthma is treated. These drugs specifically target molecules and processes linked to asthma inflammation. Monoclonal antibodies like omalizumab, mepolizumab, and benralizumab are a few examples. These medications have demonstrated astounding efficiency in lowering asthma flare-ups and enhancing lung function.

2.   **Precision   Medicine:**   Genomic advancements have made it possible to treat asthma patients individually. Healthcare professionals can optimize medicine selections and doses by assessing a patient's genetic profile and then

customizing treatment programs to meet specific needs.

3. **Mucus-Reducing Medications:** Scientists are working on drugs that can thin and thicken mucus in the airways, making it simpler to remove and lowering coughing and wheezing.

4. **Vaccines for Allergen Tolerance:** Exciting research is being done to provide vaccinations that might promote allergy tolerance. By desensitizing the immune system to common allergens, these vaccinations hope to lessen asthma symptoms brought on by allergies.

5. Telemedicine: Digital health technologies and telemedicine are becoming more and more important in the therapy of asthma. By enabling remote monitoring of asthma

symptoms, medication adherence, and virtual consultations with medical professionals, these technologies enhance patient access to care.

6. **Environmental Interventions:** Asthma trigger research has sparked the development of creative environmental treatments. As smart air purifiers and strategies to reduce allergens become more widely available, indoor settings are getting healthier.

7. **Behavioral Interventions:** Behavioral therapies, such as programs for self-management and asthma education, have shown beneficial in enhancing asthma control and lowering hospital admissions.

8. **Asthma Prevention:** A significant amount of research is devoted to preventing

asthma, particularly in young children. Studies examine variables that may affect the development of asthma, such as breastfeeding, food, and early exposure to allergens.

Hope for a World with Fewer Asthma Cases

Healthcare workers, researchers, and organizations from all around the world share the objective of lowering the incidence of asthma and enhancing asthma management. Here are several causes for optimism for a future with fewer incidences of asthma:

1. **Increased Awareness:** Early diagnosis and improved control of the illness are the results of more understanding of the risk

factors, symptoms, and therapy options for asthma.

2. **Preventive Measures:** Public health initiatives have placed a strong emphasis on preventative strategies that can lessen the chance of developing asthma, such as lowering exposure to allergens, air pollutants, and cigarette smoke.

3. **Improved Maternal Health:** According to research, a child's likelihood of having asthma can be affected by maternal health and prenatal variables. There is a chance that we can lower the number of children with asthma by enhancing mother health during pregnancy.

4. **Advancements in Medications:** The development of new drugs has made asthma treatment easier to control and

more widely available. These medications are more effective and have fewer adverse effects as a result of ongoing research.

5. **Environmental Interventions:** Especially for children who are at risk, improvements in minimizing environmental asthma triggers can result in better indoor and outdoor settings.

6. **Vaccination Strategies:** As research advances, allergen tolerance vaccinations may prove to be an effective preventative measure, lowering the prevalence of allergic asthma.

7. **Telemedicine and Digital Health:** The broad use of telemedicine and digital health tools can improve the management of asthma, particularly in underprivileged populations.

8. **Global Collaborations:** International partnerships in asthma research and care might hasten developments and increase access to high-quality care.

While these advancements provide optimism for a future with fewer incidences of asthma, it's vital to keep in mind that for many people and families, asthma still poses a serious health burden. To reduce the prevalence of asthma and enhance the quality of life for those who have it, more research, advocacy, and access to healthcare are needed.

There is cause for hope as we look to the future of asthma research and therapy. The way asthma is managed is changing as a result of developments in medicines, precision medicine, environmental interventions, and telemedicine. We are getting closer to a future where kids and families may breathe easier knowing that asthma can be properly controlled and, one day, even prevented thanks to these advancements, as well as improved awareness and preventative initiatives.

Although the road ahead may still be filled with obstacles, it is one marked by optimism, advancement, and a common dedication to bettering the lives of individuals who are impacted by asthma.

Chapter 12

Additional Resources

Families dealing with pediatric asthma must have access to trustworthy resources and assistance. An extensive list of additional resources is provided in this chapter, including a lexicon of asthma-related words, information on how to locate pediatric asthma physicians, asthma foundations, organizations, and online support groups.

Online Support Groups and Communities

Connecting with Others Facing Similar Challenges

Parents, caregivers, and children with asthma have access to helpful online forums where they may connect, exchange experiences, and get guidance from others dealing with the same issues.

Popular Online Support Groups and Communities:

1. **Asthma and Allergy Foundation of America (AAFA) Community:** The AAFA has an online forum where people who suffer from allergies and asthma may ask questions, share stories, and get assistance.

2. **Inspire Asthma and Allergy Support Group:** This Inspire online support group connects and exchanges information among individuals and families impacted by asthma and allergies.

3. **Reddit Asthma Community (r/Asthma):** On Reddit, there is a section dedicated to asthma discussions where people may

discuss the condition, share stories, ask questions, and provide support.

4. **Parents of Kids with Asthma Facebook Group:** This is a private Facebook group where parents of children with asthma can connect, exchange tips, and share stories.

5. **Kids with Asthma Instagram Community:** On Instagram, a large number of people and businesses provide instructional materials, autobiographies, and advice on pediatric asthma.

Asthma Organizations and Foundations

Key Organizations Dedicated to Asthma Advocacy and Support

Organizations and charities devoted to asthma are excellent resources for information, support, and advocacy for families with children who have asthma.

Prominent Asthma Organizations and Foundations:

1. **Asthma and Allergy Foundation of America (AAFA):** The Asthma and Allergy Foundation of America (AAFA) is a major organization that works to enhance asthma management and awareness by offering resources, educating the public, and advocating on their behalf.

2. **American Lung Association:** The American Lung Association has a multitude of materials on asthma, including details on diagnosis, management, and living with the condition.

3. **Global Initiative for Asthma (GINA):** The Global Initiative for Asthma (GINA) offers

information for healthcare professionals, patients, and caregivers as well as evidence-based guidelines for managing asthma.

4. **Asthma UK:** In the United Kingdom, Asthma UK provides comprehensive assistance for those living with asthma, including resources for children as well as parents.

5. **National Heart, Lung, and Blood Institute (NHLBI):** The NHLBI, which is part of the National Institutes of Health in the United States, provides educational resources and research updates on asthma.

Educational Resources for Learning About Asthma

For those who want to learn more about childhood asthma, how to treat it, and coping mechanisms, websites are a great resource.

Recommended Websites:

1. **KidsHealth (kidshealth.org):** KidsHealth provides asthma education articles for kids, parents, and teenagers.

2. **Asthma Kids (asthma.org.nz/kids):** Asthma Kids offers activities, films, and materials geared for children to help them understand and take care of their asthma.

3. **WebMD Asthma Center (webmd.com/asthma):** The asthma center on WebMD (webmd.com/asthma) provides a variety of articles, videos, and resources for comprehending and controlling asthma.

Glossary of Asthma-Related Terms

Understanding Asthma Terminology

For those who want to comprehend the illness and its treatment better, a dictionary of terminology linked to asthma can be a useful resource.

Common Asthma Terms:

1. **Asthma Action Plan:** An Asthma Action Plan is a written document that details how to manage asthma, including how to take medications and deal with symptoms.

2. **Bronchodilator:** A bronchodilator is a medication that relaxes the muscles in the airways and opens them up, making breathing easier.

3. **Peak Flow Meter:** A portable device that measures the greatest amount of air that a person can exhale, aiding in the monitoring of lung function.

4. **Spirometry:** A test of lung function that gauges how quickly and how much air a person can exhale.

5. **Inhaler:** An inhaler is a device that uses a spray or powder to deliver medication directly into the airways.

6. **Exacerbation:** An exacerbation is a rapid worsening of asthma symptoms that frequently calls for modifying medication or seeking medical attention.

7. **Spacer:** To guarantee optimal medication distribution and lower the chance of adverse effects, an inhaler spacer is a device that is attached to the inhaler.

8. **Allergen:** An allergen is a chemical that might cause an allergic reaction, which could result in symptoms of asthma.

9. **Wheezing:** A high-pitched whistling sound made when breathing that is frequently linked to congested airways.

10. **Triggers:** Chemicals or environmental variables that might aggravate asthma symptoms or cause asthma attacks.

Pediatric Asthma Specialists

Seeking Specialized Care for Children with Asthma

Children with asthma can be diagnosed and treated by pediatric asthma experts, such as pediatric pulmonologists and allergists.

How to Find Pediatric Asthma Specialists:

1. **Ask for Referrals:** Primary care doctors can refer patients to pediatric asthma specialists.

Chapter 13

Recap of Key Takeaways

Understanding Childhood Asthma

We have looked at a number of areas of childhood asthma in this guide, including:

1. **What is Asthma:** Asthma is a chronic respiratory disorder. The symptoms of asthma, which include wheezing, coughing, and shortness of breath, are caused by inflammation, constriction, and increased production of mucus in the airways.

2. **Prevalence:** Millions of people worldwide suffer from asthma, a prevalent illness in children. It comes in different degrees of severity and can manifest at any age.

3. **Triggers:** Exercise, allergies, respiratory infections, and environmental factors like air pollution and cigarette smoke can all cause asthma symptoms.

4. **Diagnosis:** A patient's medical history, physical examination, allergy testing, and lung function tests are all used to make the diagnosis.

5. **Management:** Creating an asthma action plan, taking prescription medications as directed, avoiding triggers, and scheduling routine check-ups with medical professionals are all important aspects of effective asthma management.

6. **Prevention:** Vaccinations, school accommodations, reducing triggers, making your house asthma-friendly, and routine

check-ups are all effective ways to avoid asthma attacks.

7. **Emergency Care:** It's critical to know when to seek emergency treatment for a kid experiencing a severe asthma attack in order to protect their safety and well-being.

8. **Future of Asthma:** Ongoing research indicates that asthma treatment, precision medicine, and preventative measures will advance.

9. **Resources:** A dictionary of asthma-related words, online forums, asthma organizations, websites, and pediatric asthma experts are some of the resources available to families living with childhood asthma.

Encouragement for Families Dealing with Childhood Asthma

Although managing childhood asthma can be difficult, it's important to keep in mind that you're not alone. Millions of families are facing comparable challenges all over the world. Here is some inspiration for those dealing with asthma in children:

1. **You're Strong:** You've already shown that you have these qualities by asking for advice and assistance. Managing childhood asthma requires strength and resiliency.

2. **Advocacy Matters:** One of the most crucial roles you can play in advocating for your child's health. To ensure that your child receives the care and support they require, act as an advocate at school, with

healthcare providers, and in your community.

3. **Communication is Key:** Open and constant communication with healthcare professionals is essential. Don't be afraid to voice your concerns, ask for clarifications, or ask questions about how to manage your child's asthma.

4. **Support is Available:** You and your child can navigate the difficulties of asthma with the aid of a wide range of resources, including online communities and organizations dedicated to the condition.

5. **Take It One Step at a Time:** Asthma management is a process, so it's acceptable to take things one step at a time. Celebrate modest successes and keep in mind that advancement is frequently gradual.

6. **Education is Empowerment:** The more you know about managing asthma in children, the more empowered you will be to do so. Knowledge is an effective management tool for asthma.

7. **Your Child's Well-Being is the Priority:** The most important thing to keep in mind is that your child's well-being comes first. Most children with asthma can lead active, healthy lives with the right asthma management.

The Importance of Ongoing Management and Communication

Childhood asthma is a chronic condition that requires ongoing management. Families, medical professionals, and educational institutions must continue to pay attention to it and work together. Here are some reasons why ongoing management and communication are so important:

1. **Asthma is Dynamic:** Because asthma symptoms and triggers are dynamic, it's crucial to have regular check-ups and communicate with your doctor in order to modify your asthma action plan.

2. **Medication Adherence:** Maintaining asthma control requires regular compliance with prescribed medications. Maintaining management enables the proper and efficient use of medications.

3. **Environmental Changes:** As kids advance in their education, their environments may change. The establishment of asthma accommodations can be facilitated by

regular communication with schools and teachers.

4. **Age and Development:** As kids get older, they may be better able to control their asthma on their own. Maintaining management encourages kids to take more charge of their health and supports this development.

5. **Prevention:** Vaccinations and asthma prevention strategies can be discussed during routine check-ups with medical professionals.

6. **Emergency Preparedness:** Being ready for emergencies related to asthma is a continuous process. It is crucial to regularly review the asthma action plan and make sure that all caregivers are familiar with it.

Looking Ahead to a Healthier Future

Regarding the future, there are causes for hope in the field of pediatric asthma:

1. **Advancements in Treatment:** Ongoing research is resulting in novel treatment alternatives, such as precision medicine and biologics, which provide promise for more focused and efficient management of asthma.

2. **Prevention Strategies:** Asthma prevention research is progressing, with an emphasis on vaccinations, early-life interventions, and environmental regulations to lower the risk of asthma.

3. **Education and Awareness:** Raising awareness and educating people about pediatric asthma is helping to improve early diagnosis, lessen stigma, and provide

families with the tools they need to properly manage their child's illness.

4. **Support Networks:** To establish robust support systems for families coping with children's asthma, advocacy groups, online forums, and medical professionals are collaborating.

5. **Patient Empowerment:** As they become older, kids with asthma may take a more active role in their own treatment, learning how to manage their own health and becoming advocates for it.

6. **Inspiration:** People are inspired by the success stories of those who overcame the difficulties associated with childhood asthma and accomplished amazing feats.

In closing, despite the difficulties associated with childhood asthma, it is a condition that can be successfully managed with the proper knowledge, resources, and support. Families with children who have asthma should anticipate a better future for their children by cooperating, staying well-informed, and advocating for the best care available.

Conclusion

Breathing Easy – A Journey of Hope

This book, "Breathing Easy: A Parent's Guide to Managing Kids' Asthma," set us on a path of education, direction, and optimism. Our goal has been to arm you with the tools and knowledge you need to navigate this journey with confidence and resilience, from the time you found that your kid had asthma to researching the most recent developments in asthma research and treatment.

We examined important subjects along the way, from comprehending the basics of asthma and identifying its symptoms to adopting a positive outlook and establishing objectives for your child's future. We investigated the complexities of medication administration, the development of asthma-friendly surroundings, and the development of a caring community of family members and medical professionals. Our goal was to give you a thorough resource that not only arms you with useful tips but also motivates you with tales of kids who have triumphed despite the difficulties associated with having asthma.

We hope that you will feel upbeat and empowered when you finish this book's last chapter. Even while asthma may provide difficulties, it is not an insurmountable barrier. Every child with asthma has power and potential, as is attested to by the triumph and resiliency tales presented here.

Remember that you are not navigating this path alone. There is a large group of parents, relatives, medical professionals, and researchers who are committed to helping kids with asthma. Reach out to them for advice, share your experiences with them, and take solace in the knowledge that you are working together to make a difference in the lives of children with asthma.

As we consider the future, we are filled with optimism. The landscape of asthma care is constantly changing as a result of improvements in research and therapy. Your dedication to your child's well-being is an essential component of this goal for a future with fewer occurrences of asthma and better treatment.

As you proceed, keep in mind that you are nourishing your child's potential as well as controlling their asthma. There are chances for development, resiliency, and success every day. The best gifts you can give your child on this path are your love, support, and perseverance.

We appreciate you giving us the opportunity to assist you on your journey to "Breathing Easy" and wish you and your kid a future full of health, happiness, and limitless opportunities.

Sincere regards,

Dr. George K. Shelley

Books By The Author

1. Peptic Ulcer Disease: A Holistic Guide to Peptic Ulcer Disease Treatment, Herbal Remedies, Essential Diet Menus, and Lifestyle Strategies for Prevention, Recovery, and a Healthy Stomach

Printed in Great Britain
by Amazon

41658545R00116